Birthing
PAINS

by
BONNIE BAKER

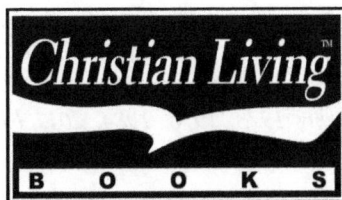

Largo, MD
USA

Christian Living Books, Inc.
P. O. Box 7548
Largo, MD 20792
christianlivingbooks.com
We bring your dreams to fruition.

ISBN Paperback 9781562293161
ISBN Electronic Version 9781562293178

Photographs by Pat McDowell

Printed in the United States of America

DEDICATION

I would like to thank my Lord and Savior Jesus Christ for inspiring me to write this book about all that I have gone through and how he healed me through it all.

But he was wounded for our transgressions, he was bruised for our iniquities: the chastisement of our peace was upon him; and with his stripes we are healed. (Isaiah 53:5)

CONTENTS

I am honored to be asked to share in this book *Birthing Pains* because I know this great, powerful woman of God personally. She is one of my God-daughters. I have observed her walk with God down through the years. It is obvious that she lives close to Him because He rewards her faithfulness with miracle, after miracle, after miracle.

Her first three books are riveting as they outline her life story. It's hard to wrap your head around the fact that this woman, small and dainty in stature, has gone through seemingly unbearable experiences prior to God coming into her life. No one person should have to suffer the things she has experienced. Yet, she came through it strong as a giant, seasoned, and now able to share testimonies and divine, supernatural, mind blowing revelation to vast audiences in churches, halls and auditoriums around the country.

In this powerful book, Evangelist Baker focuses on the importance and value of holding on in the midst of adversity. This book is filled with solid documentation of the favor of God that has been extended to her, especially the experience of crossing over to the other side, getting a glimpse of

Heaven and coming back with the ability to let us know that Heaven is real.

So, take my word for it; there is no way you can begin reading this book with any doubt, fear, or unbelief and finish it feeling the same. I visualize in the spirit right now, that as you read it, faith will begin to take legs and walk. I'm reminded of this scripture:

> Now when Jesus heard this, He was amazed at him, and turned and said to the crowd that was following Him, "I say to you, not even in Israel have I found such great faith as this man's. (Luke 7:9 AMP)

Because of her testimony, many have repented and given their hearts to God.

Evangelist Esther V. Smith
World renown author, gospel recording artist
International Gospel Center
Ecorse, MI

INTRODUCTION

Evangelist Bonnie Baker is a powerful woman of God, who has been chosen by God to be an ambassador. She is an accredited representative of Christ, tested and proven in the kingdom of God, and sent by the Lord to be a witness. Evangelist Baker continues to position herself to be used of God, to win many souls to the Kingdom of God.

> We are therefore Christ's ambassadors, as though God were making his appeal through us. We implore you on Christ's behalf: Be reconciled to God. (2 Corinthians 5:20 NIV)

I have witnessed God's overhaul in Evangelist Baker's life in so many areas. She is indeed a walking miracle and testimony before and for the Lord our God. The enemy has afflicted her many times. However, on every occasion, the Lord brought her into a wealthy place in Him and always a sure victory.

> If we suffer, we shall also reign with him: if we deny him, he also will deny us. (2 Timothy 2:12)

She is an Evangelist, Minister, Prophet, prayer warrior, and intercessor for the people of God. She is able to pray you through those HARD places, those barren seasons of heavy testing, and those times of trouble.

It is my honor and privilege to introduce this latest book to you. If you've had an opportunity to read one of her other books then you are already familiar with this great, anointed, best selling author's work.

God has allowed Evangelist Baker to experience the onslaught of the enemy in every area of her life. Chapter after chapter, God brought her out of horrific tests and trials. At the same time, He was upholding her with His right hand of righteousness, saying to the enemy, "This far and no farther." Nobody but God can get the glory for the victory given to Evangelist Baker. The weapon was formed but it couldn't prosper because of her relationship with Him.

> The angel of the LORD encampeth round about them that fear him, and delivereth them. Many are the afflictions of the righteous: but the LORD delivereth him out of them all. (Psalm 34:7,19)

So, prepare to be encouraged, enlightened, empowered and strengthened as you embark upon another masterpiece. Your faith will begin to leap in your spiritual womb concerning many of the petitions and prayers you have before the throne of the Lord our God.

Purchase one of these books for a friend, a family member, anyone you know who is going through tribulation or needs a boost in their faith. You will be blessed by this investment.

Hattie Richardson White Hopkins
Senior Pastor
Redeeming Faith International Ministries, Inc.
Greenville, NC

Chapter 1

As I sit and wait on the Lord, I heard *Write*. I thought I was done with writing but the Lord said, *NO not yet*. So, I am here to tell my story about birthing pains and how I went through them.

> To every thing there is a season, and a time to every purpose under the heaven: A time to be born, and a time to die; a time to plant, and a time to pluck up that which is planted; A time to kill, and a time to heal; a time to break down, and a time to build up. (Ecclesiastes 3:1-3)

We all have a season for our hurts, pains, trials, and tribulation. But, can we bear the pain that will come upon us when our time comes... when hurt hits us suddenly? There is a season.

Pain is a feeling of distress, often caused by intense damager stimuli, like burning your finger, bumping your big toe, hitting your funny bone, falling down, walking into a wall, getting hit, biting your tongue, cutting your nails too low, slipping in the bathroom, breaking a bone, you name it. There is a season that we will have to endure. Will you make it to the end of your birthing pains to tell your story?

Birthing pains can define many illnesses and sicknesses in our body.

In the book of Job, his friends accuse him of sinning and doing evil. They couldn't endure his suffering. They were looking for answers, and there were none. They needed a reason for his suffering, and there was none. So, they jumped to conclusions about his suffering. If you ever spend time with a suffering friend, then you know that it is hard to remain silent and not try to give some reason "why" this had to happen. The same goes for Job's three friends, Eliphaz, Bildad, and Zophar. They told Job:

> If iniquity be in thine hand, put it far away, and let not wickedness dwell in thy tabernacles. (Job 11:14)

Can you imagine what Job was thinking when his friends accused him of sin when he did not sin? You see, the devil has to go to God and ask whether or not he can put his hands upon you. But God already knows us and therefore said:

> No temptation has overtaken you that is not common to man. God is faithful, and he will not let you be tempted beyond your ability, but with the temptation he will also provide the way of escape, that you may be able to endure it. (1 Corinthians 10:13 ESV)

THERE IS A BLESSING IN THIS

All of the tribulation was the will of God for Job. Believe it or not. I had people to say to me, "Why are you going through all this sickness? This is not your year. Have you sinned or something?" Are you kidding me? Are you for real? What!?! I just couldn't believe what people were saying.

All I could say was, "NO. I have not. There is a blessing in this."

Weeping may endure for a night, but joy cometh in the morning. (Psalm 30:5b)

I was waiting on my morning.

I was waiting on my morning. People will look at what you are going through and judge you according to what they see. But, if you can get a few people – family, friends, church members – to stand with you and be there for you when you are going through, those are the ones you need in your life.

And the LORD turned the captivity of Job, when he prayed for his friends: also the LORD gave Job twice as much as he had before. (Job 42:10)

So, we have to pray for our friends. God did give me this in my suffering: family, extended family, friends, and church members who were with me during my affliction. Job did not have that.

Then said his wife unto him, Dost thou still retain thine integrity? curse God, and die. But he said unto her, Thou speakest as one of the foolish women speaketh. What? shall we receive good at the hand of God, and shall we not receive evil? In all this did not Job sin with his lips. (Job 2:9-10)

But to know it was all God's plan and His will for Job is a revelation. If your friends are not with you when you are going through trials, then you need to rethink their friendship. Always remember that there is a blessing in it. There is a double blessing if you can go through the birthing pains to receive it.

> It is good for me that I have been afflicted; that I might learn thy statutes. (Psalm 119:71)

The greatest work one can do is to do the will of God and receive from His hand. Remember that whatever you go through, there is a purpose in it. God will use that purpose to bring deliverance in someone else's life. So, while you are going through the process and giving birth to the pain, keep before you the vision that is the promise of God to bring forth the supernatural power of God within you. There is an assignment He has for you to do.

Chapter 2

Pain is an emotional experience. It is unpleasant and associated with actual damage to the body. There are all kinds of pain. Knowing the diagnoses can be very helpful at that time. Not knowing what is causing the pain can hurt more and longer. However, when you know exactly what the medical problem is, you can be treated quickly.

Pain can go on for weeks, months, and even years. This is called chronic pain. This pain is usually due to an ongoing cause, though sometimes the cause is unknown. There are many other types of pain, like syndromes, arthritis, back pain, center pain syndromes, cancer pain, headaches, central pain syndrome, head and facial pain, muscle pain, myofascial pain, disorders of the skin, sports injuries, surgical pain, and pain that's inexplicable to the doctors. Many times, the doctors will say, "We don't know what the cause is right now. But, we are still running tests."

> Beloved, think it not strange concerning the fiery trial which is to try you, as though some strange thing happened unto you. (1 Peter 4:12)

That's where birthing your pain comes in. Pain is a sign that something has gone wrong in your body. Pain is a warning of possible danger. With pain, we seek relief and comfort for our physical bodies to be healed.

One day there will be no more crying.

THERE IS NO END TO PAIN

The Bible declares that there will be a time when there will be no more pain, sin, and death, before God. Because Jesus shed His blood on the cross, this earth will be destroyed and replaced by a new heaven and a new earth. At that time, there will be no more crying, worrying, or going through.

> And God shall wipe away all tears from their eyes; and there shall be no more death, neither sorrow, nor crying, neither shall there be any more pain; for the former things are passed away. (Revelation 21:4)

However, on this earth, right now, there is no end to pain.

> But the God of all grace, who hath called us unto his eternal glory by Christ Jesus, after that ye have suffered a while, make you perfect, stablish, strengthen, settle you. (1 Peter 5:10)

Chapter 3

Every mother on this earth can attest to having labor pain; I know I can. It is the worst pain you will ever feel. Labor pain rolls in like a train and becomes harder and harder until the baby is born. After my first child, I remember saying, "I will never have another baby!" because of the pain. However, the doctor looked at my husband and said, "They all say that." So, Dean and the doctor laughed while I laid there in severe, unbearable pain. However, as soon as I had given birth to my baby, I no longer remembered the hard labor pain. All I remember was the euphoria I felt when my baby was born into the world. I was so happy and full of joy. A lot of mothers want the baby but not the pain. A lot of prospective mothers say, "If I could just have the baby without pain, I would have children." That would be great, right? It doesn't work that way, and we have Eve to thank for the pain.

Before you get to hold your baby in your arms, you have to go through three trimesters of pregnancy.

THE FIRST TRIMESTER

Your baby's development begins soon after conception. A primitive face takes form with large dark circles for eyes. A mouth, throat, and lower jaw are developing. Ears begin to form as little folds of skin on each side of the head. Tiny buds grow into arms. Also forming are fingers, toes, brain, spinal cord, nervous system, digestive tract, and sensory organs. Bone embryo begins. Blood pumps through the main vessels.

At the third month of pregnancy, your baby is fully formed. Your baby has arms, hands, fingers, feet, toes, and can open and close its fists and mouth. Toenails are developed, and ears are formed. Teeth are forming. Reproductive organs are developed. The baby's circulatory and liver produces bile. The baby's most critical development has taken place. The chance of miscarriage drops considerably after three months. Sometimes it's not good to speak on the promise, dreams, and visions too soon until the first trimester is over or done in the spirit realm. That is true for both natural birth and spiritual birth.

THE SECOND TRIMESTER

During months four through six, your baby's fingers and toes are defined. Eyelids, eyebrows, eyelashes, nails, and hair are formed. Teeth and bones are denser. The baby can suck thumbs, yawn, stretch, and makes faces. Hair is beginning to grow on baby's head. Soft, fine, hair covers shoulders, back, and temples. You can feel the baby move as muscles are developing and the baby is exercising them. By the end of the sixth month, your baby's skin is reddish in color and wrinkled; veins are visible through the skin. Baby's finger and toe prints are visible. The eyelids part and eyes open when responding to sound.

THE THIRD TRIMESTER

During the last phase before you meet the baby, fat begins to be deposited. The baby's hearing is fully developed. The baby will continue to mature and develop body fat reserves. She's kicking more. Her brain is developing rapidly and she can now see and hear. Most internal systems are well developed. Lungs are still being matured. She can blink and close her eyes, turn her head, grasp firmly, and respond to sounds, light, and touch.

SPECIAL DELIVERY

Now, the labor pain begins. Your baby's position changes to prepare itself for delivery. The baby drops down and is usually facing down toward the birth canal. Contractions can start before and after your water breaks; your cervix starts to dilate. At this point, labor is intense. The pain is getting harder and harder to bear. You are getting angry and becoming emotional. You are looking at the baby's daddy or your husband and don't want to hear *anything* he has to say. Pain becomes uncontrollable, where you can't stand it.

Push until you get the victory.

Once your cervix has dilated to ten centimeters, it's time to push the baby down the birth canal. Once you have delivered the precious baby, you begin to feel elated. You haven't quite finished labor until you push out the placenta your baby lived in while in your womb. Now, labor is complete. The joy you feel when you hear your baby's first cry is indescribable. As you hold your baby in your arms for the first time, what a beautiful feeling that is. That's birthing pains in the natural.

Well, in the spiritual realm, you have to birth every trial and tribulation, every dream and vision that the Lord has given you that you go through, until it's fully birth and you get the victory. There is a season, "spiritual birthing pains."

> A woman when she is in travail hath sorrow; because her hour has come; but as soon as she gives delivered of the child, she remembers no more the anguish, for joy that a man is born into the world. (John 16:21)

OUR RETREAT

Chapter 4

The spiritual birthing process is not easy. I would have never imagined that I would go through what I went through. I was so happy to be going to our great women's retreat in April. That morning, as I was getting ready, all I could think was, "This is my weekend! I am looking for God to do it for me inside and out. I am going to take it easy this time and just go after God for myself."

You know, sometimes preachers need a new touch from God to renew their spirits just like other Christians. We still have to cry out to God and ask Him to do it again and again in us. I know I do. So, that's what I had planned for the retreat. I wanted to get all I could get from God. As I continued to look forward to retreat week, this scripture became real in me:

> For I know the thoughts that I think toward you, said the LORD, thoughts of peace, and not of evil, to give you an expected end. (Jeremiah 29:11)

Sometimes, it takes a painful situation to carry us into a greater dimension in God. Trials strengthen our faith and take us to a place we've never been before in God. We need to come out of our comfort zones to cry loud and spare not, telling everyone that Jesus saves and He is alive for evermore. We need to declare that He is coming soon to take His people home.

God wants to put us in the right place at the right time for Him to bless us. We don't know His ways or His thoughts. When something happens likes this, we just have to believe in His promise and trust Him to the fullest.

FACING YOUR GIANT

At the retreat on Friday night, the power of God fell. We experienced an outpouring of His Spirit. Our very own first lady was the speaker that night. She preached a message entitled, "Facing Your Giant." She told us, "Shout if you believe. Pursue, overtake, and recover all." That was the breaking point. She spoke from 1 Samuel:

> And David enquired at the LORD, saying, Shall I pursue after this troop? shall I overtake them? And he answered him, Pursue: for thou shalt surely overtake them, and without fail recover all. (1 Samuel 30:8)

She began by asking us, "What are the giants in your life?" We all have some kind of giant we have to contend with – low self-esteem, lust, envy, pride, you name it. She went on to detail seven characteristics of David:

- He was responsible
- He was obedience
- He was courageous
- He was rejected
- He had a testimony

- He was himself
- He killed his giant

When God gets behind us, we can kill our giant. David won the victory with a mere slingshot. First Lady delivered a "right now" word from God with that message. I really needed to hear that.

We were asked to come and help pray the saints through. But before I went up, I cried out to the Lord right there in my seat until he bless. Remember, I had determined I would focus on me that weekend. But, with tears in my eyes, I went up to the altar and began to pray as the Lord lead me. Many souls got set free by the power of God and testified, "I am free." That was a good night. God's power came in and blessed everyone, even me, that night.

But I obeyed the Lord.

I had told my daughter Kenyatta that I was going down for early morning prayer the next morning. However, I was feeling a little bit tired from the long week at work. I had rushed directly from work to the retreat on Friday so I decided to get a little more rest the next morning.

DON'T FORGET WHAT YOU KNOW

I made it to the next sessions, refreshed. Each speaker was excellent. The speaker from Chicago spoke, "Don't forget what you know" from Jeremiah 29:11. She continued, "Don't buy into what the devil is saying and what he says is going to happen. For every problem, there is a promise. And, God has got a plan for your life." She went on to tell us, "Don't let the giants kill you. When you mess up, doesn't God still care for you? When you don't have your testimony anymore, doesn't God still care for you? God looks, sees all and still he cares for you. Don't forget what you know. When you are doing well, life happens. If everything is going well and life comes along and messes you up, can you still stand still? Pursue, overtake, and recover all when life comes along and knocks you off your feet."

Every service was like a breakthrough service. I was getting filled up and enjoying every minute, not knowing what I was going to have to face a couple of days later. The service was so awesome that I didn't want to go back to my room. I just sat there, soaking it all up, trying to process all that I have heard that weekend. I wanted to run; I wanted to holler. I wanted to shout. But, in silence, I just sat there and listened to God and… He spoke. I just couldn't wait for the evening service. We didn't know what was going to happen. But we all were ready for what God was going to do. We all look forward to a breakthrough and advancing to another level. And, God did not disappoint. On Saturday night, a speaker from Atlanta spoke from Micah:

> Be in pain, and labour to bring forth, O daughter of Zion, like a woman in travail: for now shalt thou go forth out of the city, and thou shalt dwell in the field, and thou shalt go even to Babylon; there shalt thou be delivered; there the Lord shall redeem thee from the hand of thine enemies. (Micah 4:10)

The heart of her message was to get up and do something about your situation. When you are stuck between prophecy and the plan of God, stuck between a word and the manifestation of it, stuck between a prophecy and the manifestation of it, what do you do? When wisdom can't find you, what do you do? When you say, "I know it works, but it isn't working right now. God why? God what is next? God why am I going through this? I am not equipped for this!"

She encouraged us that God has a plan that you don't understand but you still have to bring forth the baby. Pain is necessary to bring it forth. In the process you have to push to bring forth. Yes… this pain has a purpose, so bring it forth. I know it seems like this pain has brought you down to a broken state. But wait a few minutes and watch what God is doing. After the process you are much stronger; you are much wiser; So, bear the pain and push because it's for your good. It's time to push. While you are pushing remember that this pain has a purpose. Even if it looks like it's going to take your life, it's for you to bring forth. It will bring you forth to victory. This pain is for our good.

God deposited in you before the fountain of the earth. There is a song in you that God needs to be sung. There is worship in you that God needs to receive. There is a praise in you that God deserves. There is a word in you that God wants to be spoken. There is a "yes" in you that God wants to hear. God put us in pain that only He can fix.

BUT GOD KNEW

When we hear a message, though it might be encouraging, we never think it's for *us*. Every message that weekend was about pain, endurance, perseverance. Little did they know that in two days, I was going to endure pain and bring forth. But, God knew. In fact, God knew this was going to happen to me before the fountain of the earth was formed.

The glory of God was all over that meeting. It was like God, Himself, came down and walked all around putting His arms around each and every one of us. The alter call was packed; The power of God was so high; So, I decided to work the altar and pray for everyone that God lead me to, and it was many. I didn't even feel weak. It was like Jesus jumped into my body and put my flesh at the foot of the cross. We were running, crying, shouting and calling on the name of Jesus. Some people were out on the floor praising God, up against the wall, heads lying down on top of the table, where ever there was a place, we found a spot. Everyone in the building got a touch from God.

On Saturday night, as I began to hug different ones, I made my way to Kenyatta and just began to pray for her as I hugged her. She didn't want to let me go so I continued to pray for her for a while. That night she told my friend, Evangelist Gloria Burton that she saw in the spirit me having a stroke and that's why she held on to me for so long. She didn't want to let me go or for me to have to go through pain. Two days later, when it happened, Evangelist Burton didn't tell me about it until nine months later. I don't know why Evangelist Burton took so long to tell me.

Let me tell you about Kenyatta. She is definitely a praying woman of God. Don't take the way she acts and plays around for granted. She seeks the Lord. Between the ages of fourteen and seventeen, the Lord would often use her to pray and prophesy over all of us. She would wake us up to tell us "Thus said the Lord..." His power is still upon her today.

After the Saturday night service was over, I still didn't feel weak while the power of God was still there. I was praising Him all the way back to my room. Once in my room, though, I started to feel a little weak. I thought it was because I had prayed for so many people.

I couldn't go to sleep. I just wanted to praise the Lord saying, "Yes Lord. Yes Lord. Yes Lord. For the longest time. I remember falling asleep really late. When I got to church on Sunday morning I was feeling great. Once again, God moved in the service. The power of God was there. He used our Pastor again. The over flow from the retreat was there and the power of God was strong. I prayed for one person that day and just nursed because it was my Sunday to serve.

A WORD FROM THE LORD

One of the Evangelists from Chicago asked me if she could pray for me. I said yes. She said, "God said that because I had prayed for so many people and obeyed Him that He was going to bless me. God said that you have not seen what He is going to do in your life. The Glory and His anointing will rest upon you. This is just the beginning of how God is going to use you." She continued to speak what God was revealing to her and it was so powerful. I went out under the power of God. When I got up, I was still feeling good and thanking God for what He had said to me. I got me another shout in and was feeling really high in the Lord.

Once we went home, I went right to bed still saying, "Yes Lord. Have Your way. I couldn't stop saying it. The next morning when I got up for work, I was still feeling good and praising God. I began to say, "Thank You, Lord." with singing and praising God in my heart. Now, I know that God was preparing me for what was about to change my life for real. I went from a life of health to taking every kind of medicine there is... a life that knocked me off my feet.

> Speaking to yourselves in psalms and hymns and spiritual songs, singing and making melody in your heart to the Lord. (Ephesians 5:19)

THE STROKE

Chapter 5

Monday, April 4, 2016 at about 8:30 AM, I was at work. I felt my hand tingling and getting numb. I tried to shake it off and didn't think much of it. I did tell my co-worker about it. Around 2:00 PM, I felt worse and worse. My face, arm and foot began to tingle and feel numb. It was tingling really badly and all on the right side. I couldn't take it anymore. I then asked my co-work what she thought it all meant.

I began to think, "What is this? I am not feeling so good after that great move of God. But, I am still feeling the power of God all over me!" You see, you don't have to sin are do any evil for sickness to attack you. I was just coming out of a weekend retreat where God meet us there in every service. Job didn't sin or do no evil either yet his friends believed that he had.

When I got off work, I called my husband to tell him what was going on. Right away he said, "Call your doctor!" I did and she sent me right to the emergency room in West Bloomfield MI. When we got there they took me right back and ran all kinds of test.

MINI?

The diagnosis was a TIA, Transient Ischemic Attack which is commonly referred to a as a "mini-stroke." The doctors told me that it is more of a "warning stroke." TIA is caused by a clot and does have the same signs and symptoms of a stroke. The only difference between a stroke and TIA is that with TIA the blockage is transient.

I was in so much pain. I felt weakness and numbness in my face, arm, leg and foot, all on my right side. However, the doctor kept saying I didn't have a stroke and it was just a TIA. Three days later, they sent me home. I was still in a lot of pain. Those same areas were numb and tingling more and more. So, I didn't want to be sent home.

The very next day, I was right back in the emergency room with the same symptoms. As I laid there, I could feel the numbness and tingling getting worse and worse. At some point, I knew something felt different in my body. I told my baby daughter, LaChisa, to let the nurse know that I was getting worse. I could feel something coming up from my foot to my leg and on up, and it was coming up really fast. I couldn't feel my face, hand, foot, or my leg any more as the pain got worse. The nurse came in and said the doctor had ordered an MRI and that they will come and get me soon. The doctor has also prescribed pain medication.

The strokes that I had happened right there in the emergency room as I laid there in pain. We waited for over seven hours for the MRI. They gave me some pain medicine to make me comfortable. At about 5:00 AM, they came and got me. By then, I couldn't feel anything on my right side. I could tell that something serious was happening in my body.

WAIT…WHAT?

At 7:30 AM, the doctors came in and told me that I had in fact had a stroke and it hit deep in the back of my head. I was messed up after that because I laid there for seven hours and they did nothing. Maybe it was because I was there the night before. Perhaps they didn't believe me. Maybe they thought it was another TIA. But, at that point I was too through… like for real! This was Friday morning.

I just could not believe it. I tried to open my hand but it was paralyzed. I couldn't lift my leg. I began to cry, cry, cry, cry, weep and cry. I was hurt… very hurt… and I just didn't understand why this happened. "I had a stroke!" Every time I thought about *that*, I cried. As I write this book, I am reliving it all over again, and it's very painful. But, never once did I get mad or angry at God. I began to think about all the services during the retreat and all the messages. After all, all I *could* do was lay there and think. I thought about what God had spoken to me on Sunday morning. I remembered the way God used me to pray for so many people. I wondered whether or not I had overextended myself… taxed my body… over did it. I reminded myself that God will not put any more on you than you can bear. I thought that for this purpose God will get the glory. Oh my God did He get the glory. Just wait until the end of this testimony. Despite all that, I was just hurt. I could not understand how this could follow that great and powerful weekend at the women's retreat. By now, everyone was praying:

> And all things, whatsoever ye shall ask in prayer, believing, ye shall receive. (Matthew 21:22)

> And this is the confidence that we have in him, that, if we ask any thing according to his will, he heareth us. (1 John 5:14)

My sister Pastor Hattie Hopkins and her husband Dr. Frederick Hopkins in North Carolina often fasted and prayed for me. They had every one at their church, Redeeming Faith International Ministries in Greenville, North Carolina, praying. All of her affiliated churches were praying in the surrounding areas and out of town. My sister Barbara and her husband, all my family and friends were praying. My church family was praying. Nevertheless, God still allowed it to happen. And… He can do that because He is God and beside Him there is none other.

God still allowed it to happen.

I was reminded why birthing pains are so hard… the pain is heavy and unbearable. All day Friday I was still messed up from this happening. That evening, my husband called our Pastor and told him about it. Pastor said, I'm coming. The devil *is* a liar!"

> Therefore I say unto you, What things soever ye desire, when ye pray, believe that ye receive them, and ye shall have them. (Mark 11:24)

The next morning as prayer was still going up from everywhere, my sister Pastor Hopkins said they stayed in prayer all day and night for God to work a miracle. My brother, Prophet Nathaniel Richardson in Greenville North Carolina said he saw in the spirit as he was praying that he came in the room and prayed for me and I got up and started to shout.

My Pastor and First Lady walked in the room the next morning. I looked up and said, "Bless you." Now, I want you to know we had just came out of a John the Baptist, devil chasing, foot stomping, women's retreat and the power of God was still present. We talked and Pastor said, "Let's pray." He began to rub all up and down my side, my hand, my foot and knee.

First Lady was on one side with all of the power from the women retreat all over her. Pastor was on the other side. The Lord used them as they prayed and prayed. With prayer still going on in North Carolina and New York and all the churches that were praying... the devil *had* to go. The devil meant it for evil but, God turned it around.

OH MY GOD!

All of a sudden... my hand began to open up out of the paralysis position. I started crying, hollering, and screaming. I lifted it all the way up and it was open. Oh my God... all the way open! Glory to God. Praise the Lord. Hallelujah! So, Pastor said, "I feel like praying for everyone in here." I was thinking, "Well... finish with me first because God was moving on my behalf and I didn't want Him to stop!" Now *that* was something to see – all three of us saw it unfold right before our eyes.

> The effectual fervent prayer of a righteous man availeth much. (James 5:16b)

I then held up my foot and began to move my toes. I bent my knee. I was so happy to know God did a miracle right there in the hospital bed for me. I was doing everything I couldn't do before. I almost jumped out the bed. I told them to go get the nurse so that I can get up. I was hooked up to everything and I said under hook me *please*.

When my husband and Kenyatta arrived, and saw me, they just didn't believe what they were seeing. And I asked Dean to unhook me from all this stuff so that I can praise the Lord and shout. He said, Wow! I can't believe this! I just wanted to give Him praise and thank Him for what He had done. The nurse came in and saw me with my hands up and praising the Lord.

She said, "What happened?"

I said, "God moved."

She said, "Did this *just* happen?"

I said, "Yes it did!"

She ran out of my room and told everyone she could find. She brought the doctors in.

They asked the same thing, "What happened!?!"

So, I said it again… "God moved. See what I can do now?"

They said, "With this type of stroke, you shouldn't be doing all this… Not this quick or this soon."

I said, "What? God is a good God. Yes He is!"

So, the doctors start running more tests and every one of them came back normal. As of result of having the stroke, my right side is always cold from my face to my toe. "But, GOD."

> No weapon that is formed against thee shall prosper; and every tongue that shall rise against thee in judgment thou shalt condemn. This is the heritage of the servants of the LORD, and their righteousness is of me, saith the LORD. (Isaiah 54:17)

God is so good and almighty. I am giving Him all the glory because my mouth is not twisted. My hand is not in a paralyzed position. My leg and foot are not twisted. My body is not paralyzed. I am not in a wheel chair, debilitated. I praise God for that. I praise Him every time I think about the way I could have ended up. I pray for everyone I see in that state. To know that He spared me from being the way I *could* have been.

> Ye are of God, little children, and have overcome them: because greater is he that is in you, than he that is in the world. (1 John 4:4)

Hallelujah, thank you JESUS. Many have called me the "miracle woman." But I call myself Bonnie a servant of the most high God. I will serve Him until I die. Without Him, I am nothing. Without Him, I can do nothing.

> Again I say unto you, that if two of you shall agree on earth as touching any thing that they shall ask, it shall be done for them of my Father which is in heaven. (Matthew 18:19)

Chapter **6**

He gives power to the faint; and to them that have no might he increaseth strength. (Isaiah 40:29)

I went from the hospital right to rehabilitation facility to get physical therapy. I was there for almost a month. Therapy was twice a day. I was during so good in therapy that other patients thought I was a visitor. Others asked, "How is it that you had a stroke but doing what the therapist is telling you to do so well?"

I didn't look like I had had a stroke. And that was nobody but God. My heart went out to every patient there. I began to pray for the other patients. Some were paralyzed all the way down on one side and couldn't move. Some were in wheel chairs, walking with walker, using canes, bedfast. Others couldn't talk. Some couldn't walk. Many had mouths that were badly twisted. Some had sores everywhere on their bodies. That could have been me. If the Lord was not on my side.

It was just bad. I didn't want to be there. I kept thinking that there has to be a reason why I am here. There were all different kind of sicknesses there. It was just a lot to handle.

Ephesians 6:10 declares, "Be strong in the Lord and in the power of his might." So, I stayed in prayer for them. I laid awake many nights, looking up in the ceiling, praying for the people of God, praying for healing in their bodies, soul and minds, asking Him to heal all sickness and disease. I had a chance to witness to everyone who came to my room telling them about the love of Jesus.

I remember this one lady in therapy keep crying out, "I can't do this. It hurt so bad." Right there, tears began to fill my eyes as I watched her say that over and over again. All I could do was cry. Her therapist was very gentle with her. My therapist asked me, "Is everything OK? Are you alright? I know it's hard." As tears rolled down my face, I said, "Can I go back to my room because the Lord had blessed me to look as if I haven't even had a stroke." I just couldn't stand to see other patients looking like that. We all had had strokes and were in rehab for recovery. Some days were better than others.

> For I will restore health unto thee, and I will heal thee of thy wounds, saith the LORD. (Jeremiah 30:17a)

COMING OUT OF MY PAIN

They gave me a wheel chair and I came up out of that. They gave me a walker and I came up out of that. They gave me a cane and I didn't really need that. I am walking, talking, lifting my hands and giving God all the glory. Many stroke patients don't come out that way. I am so grateful to God. He did it and only Him.

I was discharged and then had in-home therapy for a month. After that, I was going to therapy four times a week.

Now, I only go two times a week. I remember my mother having many small strokes before she had a major one that left her paralyzed on one side. She couldn't walk and her arm was in a paralyzed position. Gangrene set in her big toe and up her leg. So, her leg was amputated all the way up to her thigh. As my brother, Deacon Armie, picked her up to put her on the couch while I was there visiting, she said, "Boy don't hurt my leg." But she didn't have that leg anymore. Oh my God. I miss her and Daddy so much. I can barely talk about this. I'm in tears and crying now. I just miss them so much. I've got to stop now. I will be back after I regroup...

I had a talk with Jesus and feel better now. I am back! I got it together. She is now with Jesus, Daddy, her three sons Jack, Clarence, Alexander, her family, my nine children (three sons and six daughters) and so many, many, many more... too many to name.

> We are confident, I say, and willing rather to be absent from the body, and to be present with the Lord. (2 Corinthians 5:8)

In July 2016, we lost our brother Alexander. That was very hard because we were the last ones at home with mom and dad. I have so many stories of him and my other two brothers Deacon Armie and Prophet Nathaniel. But I digress...

BACK TO BACK

After I got back from Alexander's funeral, the next day, I walked onto the back of my granddaughter's heel and broke two of my toes! They were split wide open on guess which side... my right side... the same side I had the stroke on. They are still bigger than normal to this day. I began to think about my first book *Then and Now* when everything was happening back to back… like a roller coaster… one thing after another. It felt just like that. I thought, "What could be next? But, I was reminded of the scripture:

What could be next?

But he knoweth the way that I take: when he hath tried me, I shall come forth as gold. (Job 23:10)

Oh yes! I am waiting for my blessing. It's coming. So, remember; if you are going through hard tests and trials, know this for sure "it's a blessing in it." Just go through the process and victory is yours.

PASSING OUT

Chapter 7

On the morning of September 6, 2016 at 9:30 AM, I pulled up to my house, got out of the car, and collapsed... unconscious until I got in the ambulance. My daughter and her friend were parking behind me. So, she ran and caught me before I hit the ground. I was taken by ambulance to St. Mary Mercy Hospital in Livonia, Michigan.

At the hospital, I was confused and didn't know any one. My blood sugar was very high. After a lot of tests was run, I was sent by ambulance to Henry Ford Hospital in West Bloomfield, Michigan. I was there for four days. They ran every test you can think. Doctors were saying it's this and that but it was none of anything they initially thought. All tests came back negative. They had no answers. I was sent home not knowing why I passed out.

On the evening of December 31, 2016 about 4:00 PM, I was having a great day out doing a little shopping Friday before church on Saturday night. I put out my clothes. I was ready for a blessed night... I was happy to bring in the New Year with family, friends and church family.

I started feeling a little bad in Walmart. I didn't think much of it and continued to shop. My friend and her daughter were with me. They noticed it and told me to sit down while they finished getting what I wanted. I agreed and took a seat. Once we got to the car, I noticed that I was getting a bit confused. Getting into the car, I almost fell, so they both helped me into the car.

Inside the car, I looked up in the sky and saw my mother. She was just smiling at me. So, I began to wave at her. She then turned and began to leave. So, I asked why she was leaving and why did she come. I was speaking out loud. So, on the way home, I was told that I became more disoriented and didn't know where I was.

They got me home and called for my husband to come downstairs to check me out. He came down and checked my vital signs. My blood pressure was very high. He tried to give me my night medicine but I didn't want to take it. I was shaking my head and would not allow him to put the pills in my mouth.

NO RESPONSE

I didn't know anyone and was asking, "Who is this little boy?" speaking of Ivan, my grandson, the son we always wanted. Dean called 911. I had passed out and was unresponsive. The paramedics began to do a sternum rub and everything else that they could do to wake me up but they got no response.

I was transported by ambulance to St. Mary Mercy Livonia Hospital. The ER doctors did the same things to try to wake me up. They ran every test they could to find out what the problem was. But, they didn't find anything.

All the tests they run came back negative. They checked to see if I had, had another stroke and I had not.

So, they admitted to the Intensive Care Unit because I was still unconscious and unresponsive. I was told that they too did the sternum rubs to try and wake me.

Some might ask, "What is a sternum rub?" According to Judith Lower in *Facing Neuro Assessment Fearlessly*, "It is a pain stimulus technique used by medical personnel for assessing the consciousness level of a person who is not responding to normal interaction, voice commands or gentle physical stimuli such as shaking of the shoulders." Two weeks after I was discharged my chest was still red, tender and sore. Back to the ICU...

The doctors did not let my husband and children come back to see me until an hour later because I was still unresponsive after I was admitted to the hospital. I still was when they did eventually come back to see me. My daughters, Kenyatta and Chantal, began to call the family to let everyone know to be praying. My sister Barbara, husband Shelly and their church family in Tennessee were praying and calling. My brother James and his wife Ora in Florida were praying and calling. My husband talked to our Pastor that night on the phone and Pastor said, "She's going to wake up."

Everyone was worried, worried, worried and didn't know if I was coming back or not. My family stayed and slept in the hospital all that night and the next day. Dr. and Pastor Hopkins were on it – calling everyone to go into intercessory prayer and not let up, saying the devil is a liar.

"You won't have another one."

She told me after I got out of the hospital that she saw me slipping away; she said she went into her bedroom and began to tell the devil, "You won't have another one of my family members… not another one of my siblings… not my sister Bonnie."

THE OTHER SIDE

As they all continued in prayer, I was still out and unresponsive. While, I was out I began to defy gravity and walk towards these super bright, powerful lights I saw. As I was walking and floating to the lights, they got brighter and brighter. I was trying so hard to get there and go behind the lights because you could see that something very, very beautiful was on the other side. That happened three times.

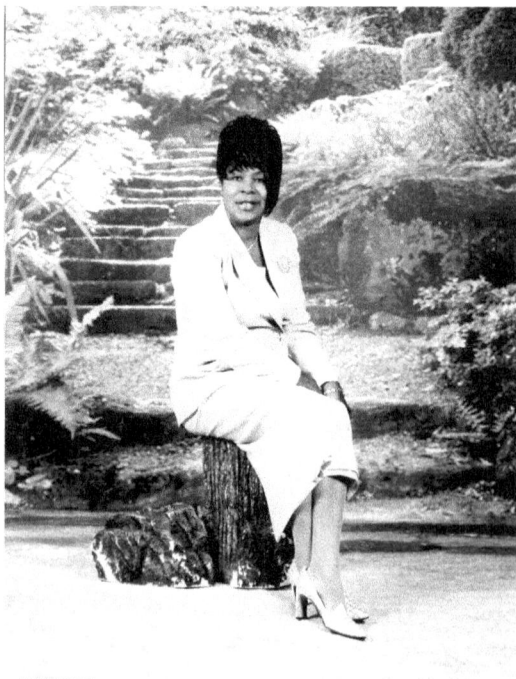

As I was looking back down on my family, the look on their faces made me sad as they wanted me to wake up and I couldn't. I took a close look at each one, where they were sitting, and how they were worried and wondering if I was coming back or not. Dean was sitting right beside me in the bed. The girls were on the coach. My friend and her daughter were at the end of the bed. I was wondering where I was. Then, it hit me. I was on my way to Glory, floating on gravity to the super bright, bright powerful lights. I knew I was out of my body. I didn't want to leave them...

And at one point, I heard Ivan calling me, "Granny, Granny." I began to think about all my family, my extended family and friends. I thought, "If I go over to the other side, I will miss them. I do want to see my Lord and Savior Jesus Christ, my family, nine children and everyone else there on the other side."

I turned back toward the lights and then I heard a voice. I began to go toward that voice. That voice began to speak to me and say, "Come closer. Come closer my daughter." Then, I realized, that it was Jesus talking to me. He began to tell me, "I'm coming soon. We are now in the days of when things will start to change. He was speaking, almost verbatim from the scriptures:

> Jesus answered: "Watch out that no one deceives you. For many will come in my name, claiming, 'I am the Messiah,' and will deceive many. You will hear of wars and rumors of wars, but see to it that you are not alarmed. Such things must happen, but the end is still to come. Nation will rise against nation, and kingdom against kingdom. There will be famines and earthquakes in various places. All these are the beginning of birth pains. (Matthew 24:4-8 NIV)

Other things were said but I cannot remember every word. The second time, He called my name and said, "Bonnie. Bonnie. Come closer. Come closer." He was standing on the banks of Heaven and showing me just a tiny glimpse. I cannot even describe it. But, as He continued to call, I started thinking, "Am I dead? Am I about to cross over into Glory?" I looked back at my family. I didn't want to leave them. I put my face in my hands and held my head down and became so very afraid. I really thought I was on the other side. When I held my head up, He started talking to me. "Many people will not get a chance to see this as you have."

Reconciliation is always at the heart of God. He is ever using every available means to get people the message. What He gave me is this: "Tell everyone that time is winding up. I am soon to come. Get your house in order. Seek me while I may be found today because tomorrow is not promised. You can be here today and gone tomorrow."

I had had an out of body experience before, in 2001. I describe it in Chapter 10 of *Then and Now*. But I live to live again and to see Jesus. To get that close to the other side and have to come back is an indescribable experience. I tell you… to make it in is your gain. To be close to Him is where I want to be.

> Seek ye the Lord while he may be found, call ye upon him while he is near. (Isaiah 55:6)
>
> O Lord my God, I cried unto thee, and thou hast healed me. (Psalm 30:2)
>
> He sent His word, and healed them, and delivered them from their destructions. (Psalm 107:20)

Chapter **8**

As much prayer was still going up in and out of town, the doctors stated that I was completely unconsciousness, unresponsive and not responding to anything... not even to pain. I was basically in a comatose state.

To me though, being out was the most wonderful feeling I had ever experienced. I was talking with Jesus, floating around, looking at the big bright, powerful lights. As I looked down at my family I tried to say something to them but they could not hear me talking to them. I called Dean's name so many times saying, "Hey! I am up here!" He didn't even look up.

That's when I began to become a little sad, when none of my family heard me talking to them. I said to myself, "Have I died?" But because of the conversation I was having with Jesus, I knew I was out of my body. But, I knew I was not out of the body to be present with the Lord yet.

For the Lord himself shall descend from heaven with a shout, with the voice of the archangel, and with the trump of God: and the dead in Christ shall rise first: Then we which are alive and remain shall be caught up together with them in the clouds, to meet the Lord in the air: and so shall we ever be with the Lord. (1 Thessalonians 4:16-17)

For yourselves know perfectly that the day of the Lord so cometh as a thief in the night. (1 Thessalonians 5:2)

I believe God took me through that to tell his people what He said: "To get ready. I am coming. Prepare ye. Prepare ye. I am coming back. Get ready. Remember the Ten Commandments and keep them."

"I *am* the LORD your God, who brought you out of the land of Egypt, out of the house of bondage. "You shall have no other gods before Me. "You shall not make for yourself a carved image – any likeness *of anything* that *is* in heaven above, or that *is* in the earth beneath, or that *is* in the water under the earth; you shall not bow down to them nor serve them. For I, the LORD your God, *am* a jealous God, visiting the iniquity of the fathers upon the children to the third and fourth *generations* of those who hate Me, but showing mercy to thousands, to those who love Me and keep My commandments. "You shall not take the name of the LORD your God in vain, for the LORD will not hold *him* guiltless who takes His name in vain. "Remember the Sabbath day, to keep it holy. Six days you shall labor and do all your work, but the seventh day *is* the Sabbath of the LORD your God. *In it* you shall do no work: you, nor your son, nor your daughter, nor your male servant, nor your female servant, nor your cattle, nor your stranger who *is* within your gates. For *in* six days the LORD made the heavens and the earth, the sea, and all that *is* in them, and rested the seventh day. Therefore the LORD blessed the Sabbath day and hallowed it. "Honor your father and your mother, that your days may be long upon the land which the LORD your God is giving you. "You shall not murder. "You shall not commit adultery. "You shall not steal. "You shall not bear false witness against your neighbor. "You shall not covet your neighbor's house; you shall not covet your neighbor's wife, nor his male servant, nor his female servant, nor his ox, nor his donkey, nor anything that *is* your neighbor's." (Exodus 20:2-17 NKJV)

But of that day and hour knows no man, no, not the angels of heaven, but my Father only. (Matthew 24:36)

As my family waited and waited on the doctors and specialists, watching and looking for a miracle for me to respond, wake up, say something, the day and hours began to take a toll on them.

"SHE IS GOING TO WAKE UP!"

By this time, I was told that Pastor called and said, "I am on my way and she is going to wake up." When Pastor got there, he greeted everyone and said, "You are about to witness a miracle. She going to wake up." He took one hand and my husband took the other one. They were on both sides of the bed. The Lord began to use Pastor as he prayed, "Bonnie. Bonnie. Pastor's here. Bonnie open your eyes." They say I started moving my head from side to side. That was something I hadn't done since I being admitted to the hospital.

The third time Pastor called my name, I heard someone saying, "Bonnie" in a really, really quiet voice. At that moment, I was just about to go into the bright lights. I had been trying to cross over. I knew that Glory was on the other side. But, I turned around and looked back. I saw someone there and heard my name being called. Jesus pushed me and said, "Go back!" They said my body started shaking and trembling. I jumped up off the bed as if someone had put a big electric shock in my back. Then, my eyes opened and I looked and tried to say "Pastor" but no sounds were coming out of my mouth. He said, "Devil you are a liar" then put his hand under my mouth. The Lord used him again. When he finished praying, I opened my mouth and said "Pastor, Pastor, Pastor, Pastor, Pastor" When I looked at Dean he said, "Do you know who I am?" I said "Yes Dean, Dean, Dean, Dean, Dean. Everyone began to rejoice.

Pastor said, "You all just witnessed a miracle. God is real." Some of my children had left the room to get food. They returned saying "Mommy, Mommy" rejoicing to see me, hugging me and kissing me. Kenyatta asked, "Mommy, did you see JESUS?" I told her what I saw: her grandma, the bright lights, the whole bit.

A miracle just happened.

Pastor then said, "Go get the nurses and tell them that a miracle just happened."

The nurse came in and said, "Your eyes are open. Wow! I can see your eyes. Wow. What just happened?"

"MY PASTOR PRAYED"

I said, "My Pastor prayed." I don't know if she really believed me or not. She went and got the doctors and specialist. They also said, "Wow. You are awake." They were all amazed and shocked. They said, "She just woke up. What happened again? I said, "My Pastor prayed." They said, in shock,

"Thank You, Jesus" I am here to tell you that my God is still working miracles.

I am running for my life crying loud and sparing not to tell people to come in. Jesus saves and will save you if you want to be saved.

> Jesus answered, Verily, verily, I say unto thee, Except a man be born of water and of the Spirit, he cannot enter into the kingdom of God. (John 3:5)

We have a powerful man of God here. Let's not take him for granted. My discharge papers stated Coma 3. We sit here, under all this anointing, week after week. It's like Dean said. Pastor walked in the room with Jesus with him and messed everyone up in the room... family, nurses, doctors. Everyone in the room saw a miracle unfold right before their eyes. Jesus is real.

Even the hospital had to acknowledge the miracle. My discharge papers from St. Mary Mercy Hospital state, "Patient continued to be unresponsive to verbal stimuli and had her eyes closed until the afternoon of the day of discharge. On day of discharge, Patient spontaneously woke up and became responsive as her Pastor walked in the room and called out her name." They gave God all the credit for using our Pastor that evening.

BIRTHING PAINS

Chapter 9

Spiritual birthing pains are just like... those you experience in natural birth. In a spiritual pregnancy you are carrying pain until you birth it. You have to bring forth a vision or a dream from God by seeking God, getting intimate with Him, and birthing it in the spirit realm.

When you build an intimate relationship with the Lord, He then will impregnate you with something planted in you by Him in the spirit. Dreams and visions grow and develop by travailing, praying and fasting to birth it. You must then take that vision which has been supernaturally planted in you by God, to fulfill God's promise for your life.

We as Christians in God have to stay focused on the Lord to bring forth those things that He had for us from the began of the world.

> Before I formed you in the womb I knew you, before you were born I set you apart; I appointed you as a prophet to the nations. (Jeremiah 1:5 NIV)

Before we were born He knew us and gave that to us to be birthed.

> For I know the thoughts that I think toward you, saith the LORD, thoughts of peace, and not of evil, to give you an expected end. (Jeremiah 29:11)

Wake up, dreams and visions. Come forth, dreams and visions. You are in a spiritual womb and it's time to bring you forth. Can you feel the birthing pains? It's time. Someone is about to give birth to that dream. Someone is about to give birth to that vision. Live on, dreams and visions.

I know many men and women of God, personally, who have suffered before death, birthing in the spirit what God called them to do. Let's not forget the many men and women of God in the Bible who suffered before death and some didn't die.

A PURPOSE FOR PAIN

Job's suffering was not caused by sin. Scripture tells us that Job was "blameless and upright," someone who "feared God and avoided evil." (Job1:1) Many people wonder why God allowed their loved one to suffer. Sometimes, it's not for the one that is suffering. It could be for the family of the one that is suffering. God could be trying to get their attention. Then, once God has their attention, He calls that suffering one in to Glory.

Job knew the difference between suffering and redemption. He hoped for salvation even in the midst of suffering.

> For I know that my redeemer liveth, and that he shall stand at the latter day upon the earth: And though after my skin worms destroy this body, yet in my flesh shall I see God: Whom I shall see for myself, and mine eyes shall behold, and not another; though my reins be consumed within me. (Job 19:25-27)

In some cases, the suffering servant of the Lord can bring about salvation to family that God is waiting to save or deliver from unforgiveness, hatred, drugs, and all the things that have them bound. The person that is suffering may not even know it. The person that is sick doesn't want to see their loved ones lost with no hope. They wanted to see them saved.

I had a person to ask me why God is allowing their grandmother to suffer from one sickness after another. I reply, "It's not for her suffering and sickness. It's for her family. God knows and He sees what she is going through." Many times, the family will give their life to the Lord. But, after a while they go back to their old ways and forget about God.

Birthing in pain is what we have to endure to get to the promises, dreams and visions God has had for us from the beginning of the world. The pain starts from the first trimester and continues through the final stages of pregnancy.

You have to go through a process.

Until the promise is birthed, you *have* to go through a process. There are many types of birthing pain. You can feel the birthing pains coming when it's time to be set free. The moaning and the groaning in the spirit starts. That's when you let the Holy Spirit take over your prayer so you can travail through the trials and tribulation. Birthing pains are not easy.

Your spiritual birthing could be anything that you are going through – your children, husband, wife, job, boss, church, friends, family, sickness or yourself. This scripture talks about all the flesh that has to be killed before you can walk in victory.

> Now the works of the flesh are manifest, which are these; Adultery, fornication, uncleanness, lasciviousness, Idolatry, witchcraft, hatred, variance, emulations, wrath, strife, seditions, heresies, envyings, murders, drunkenness, revellings, and such like: of the which I tell you before, as I have also told you in time past, that they which do such things shall not inherit the kingdom of God. (Galatians 5:19-21)

You have to cultivate the fruit of the spirit.

> But the fruit of the Spirit is love, joy, peace, longsuffering, gentleness, goodness, faith, meekness, temperance: against such there is no law. (Galatians 5:22-23)

To give birth to the fruit of the spirit you have to kill the works of the flesh. That stage of deliverance is the third trimester. Labor is required to get the victory over that thing in the spirit realm. You can't take spiritual birthing pains unless God is with you. Jesus prayed and asked the Father if it were possible to let this cup pass from Him. However, He ended that prayer with, "Nevertheless, not as I will, but as thou wilt."

DON'T ABORT OR MISCARRY

Many people can and will abort their spiritual birth. They just can't take the pain any more. So, they throw in the towel and have a spiritual miscarriage. They could be almost there. Because labor is hardest just before the PUSH, many times they are right on the threshold of the victory when they give up. A winner will never quit and a quitter will never win.

Jesus took every stripe. He suffered, bleed and died. On the third day He rose so that we would have eternal life in

Glory. So, we must go through our birthing pains in the spiritual realm to win every victory.

> But he was wounded for our transgressions, he was bruised for our iniquities: the chastisement of our peace was upon him; and with his stripes we are healed. (Isaiah 53:5)

I have been there many times and gave up and had to go right back through that thing again until I got the victory over it in the spirit realm. Until I learned how to birth the pain, I ended up going over and over the same things without God. It was impossible to bear. Does it hurt? Yes it does. The pain is hard. This pain hurt inside and out. You wear it on your face and you feel in down to your very core. People wear their pain on their face when they have not learned how to disguise the hurt until they can give birth to that which they are carrying in the spirit. Everyone can see a person's pain when they wear it on their face.

The bottom line is... you *have* to go through the process to come out with the victory. You *have* to labor to give spiritual birth to the promises, dreams and visions you are carrying. When a very hard trial hits you, it almost takes you out. You make it through the pain and the process with fasting and praying, crying and praying. Once you are not wearing the pain on your face or in your body then you have broken through the birthing pains. Now... you are ready to stand tall in God.

> Now unto him that is able to do exceeding abundantly above all that we ask or think, according to the power that worketh in us. (Ephesians 3:20)

As I look back over the years and reflect on my friendship with Evangelist Bonnie Baker, I am struck anew with the realization that she is a one of a kind original! Evangelist Baker has a gregarious personality, a million-dollar smile, an infectious sense of humor, and a heart of gold. She is generous to a fault, and loves to put a smile on the faces of her friends and loved ones through her giving. But, most importantly, she is a chosen woman of God, whom He is using to impact the lives of many through her amazing testimony.

Bonnie and I met over three decades ago at my family church, the International Gospel Center in Ecorse, Michigan where my late uncle, Apostle Charles O. Miles was the presiding pastor at that time. My grandparents, Deacon Leslie and Mother Mildred Poole had all but adopted Bonnie as their fourth daughter. Because of their close relationship, she became an honorary Poole in our large, close-knit family. Bonnie was indispensable to my grandparents, and couldn't have been more supportive and loving if she had been their natural born daughter. She was truly a blessing to them throughout their lives.

Bonnie has also been a tremendous blessing to me personally. In 1994, it just so happened that a home directly across the street from her became available for sale. Bonnie called me, and put me in touch with the homeowner. My credit was less than perfect at the time, but because of Bonnie's influence with the seller, I soon became a proud, first time, home owner.

Evangelist Baker and I grew as close as sisters during this time, and would visit each other often, talking for hours on end. It was during one of these conversations that she shared her riveting life story with me. She brought tears to my eyes as she recounted her incredible life on the streets, her experiences, and her narrow escapes from death. To say that Bonnie does not look like what she's been through is a gross understatement. The fact that she is still here today is nothing short of miraculous.

I have had the opportunity to hear Evangelist Baker minister countless times over the years, and the anointing that rests over her life is directly proportionate to the missteps, mishaps, and mistakes that shaped her over the years. It is amazing to witness people being delivered and set free as she ministers and pours out what God has deposited within her over the years.

> Clearly Bonnie is one of God's favorite daughters, as He is still doing amazing things in her life. Satan has desired to sift her as wheat, and has thrown everything at her except the proverbial kitchen sink. But God has taken everything the devil meant for evil, and turned them around for her good. Bonnie's set-backs have been set-ups for a richer anointing, and a higher calling on her life. I am confident that her fourth book, *Birthing Pains* will bless you richly, and restore your faith to believe God

for what seems impossible. He is waiting to do great and mighty things for you. "For with God nothing shall be impossible." (Luke 1:37)

In His Service,
Elder Felecia Poole-Harrell
City of Faith Church
West Palm Beach, Florida

I am pleased to write these words about Evangelist Bonnie Baker. *Birthing Pains* will encourage readers that God is in control. No matter how low or even how high in life you get, God is in control. Everything has a God purpose. Evangelist Bonnie Baker has discovered the excellence in praise and gives praise in every obstacle she has encountered in life.

God has brought her from a long way and she has no problem sharing her life testimony with others to help others who are facing challenges. Evangelist Baker is a woman of God who always helps others. She loves to encourage others as well as lend a helping hand where needed.

Evangelist Baker and I have been friends for years. We've worked together on several outreach programs at International Gospel Center. Jesus said, "Go ye into all the world and preach the gospel to every living creature." (Mark 16:15) Evangelist Baker has demonstrated the essence of going into the highways and the byway places like prison, nursing homes and street ministry. She has traveled the country preaching the gospel.

Evangelist Baker is the example of a second chance in life. What the devil meant for evil God turned it around for His Glory. Bonnie was faced with a near-death experience and could have walked into eternal glory. But God said, "Go back and tell my people your story."

God's grace and mercy is the reason Evangelist Baker is alive and well today. She is telling her story to bring understanding and deliverance to people who are faced with situations only God can bring them out of – *with* a testimony that only God can get the credit for.

Evangelist Raymond Tyrone Defoe
Vice President Evangelistic Department
International Gospel Center Church

ACKNOWLEDGMENTS

I would like to thank God Almighty, my Lord and savior, Jesus Christ, for inspiring me to write this book in the spur of the moment. It was not in my plans to do so, but God's.

To my husband, Willie Dean; my children, Tawana, Kenyatta and James, Chantel, and LaChisa, for all your love, support, encouragement, and being with me during all of my sickeness. You took good care of me when you knew I was in a lot of pain. I felt the love you showed me. You exceeded every expectation. I love you all very much, more than you will ever know or think.

To my grandchildren, Ivan, Ivoree and Cleah, thanks for letting me love on you and for bringing such joy to my life.

To all my brothers, James, Armie, Nathaniel and sisters, Barbara and Hattie; To my family on both sides for being with me through this – the ones in and out of town. I love you more then you will ever know.

To my sister and brother, Pastors Frederick and Hattie Hopkins, you have always been there along with your church, Redeeming Faith International Ministries, interceding for me, not letting up, calling those things as be not as though they were, speaking life, and letting the devil know he is a liar's and the father of them. I love you so much. The love of God shine upon you and bless you and your church.

To my church family in Greenville, North Carolina at Redeeming Faith International Ministries, thanks for all your prayers. I love you.

To my extended family, Mother Evans, Gladys, Bonita, Tonia, and Chrissy who have totally been there for me since I became sick, putting up with me when I was in pain, showing me how much they care, cooking, driving me to my doctor's appointments, keeping my grandchildren so I can rest. It's been too much to say. You went over and beyond the call of duty, showing love the way God say it. Thank you so much. I love you.

To my Pastor and First Lady, Pastor Marvin N. and Carolyn Miles, Wow! What can I say but you have been there for me, visiting during all my hospital stays, letting the Lord use you in demonstrating His miracle power, leaving everyone messed up as they witnessed the miracle power of God, right before their eyes. God bless you. I love you. Thank you.

To Dr. Luvenia Miles, Dr. Shirley Hathrone, my mother now Mother Mary Jordan Meeks, Mother Wilmatine Harris, Mother Patricia Defoe, Mother Alma Snowden. For all your prayer, support and many words, thank you. I love you. May God bless you.

To a very special friend, Evangelist Gloria Burton, thank you for all your encouraging words, support, love and prayer, all the times you cried and laughed with me and for being a true friend. God bless you. Thank you. I love you.

To my church family at the International Gospel Center in Ecorse MI, for all your prayers, I thank you. I love you.

To all my friends and other loved ones, I thank you for your support, prayer, love and encouragement. Bless you, in the name of Jesus.

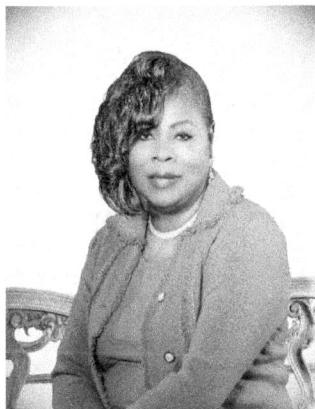

Minister Bonnie Baker was born in Vredenburgh, Alabama. She is the seventh child born to the late Jack and late Clara Richardson. She was Homecoming Queen of her high school in 1969. She always had big plans for her life. Bonnie moved to Detroit, Michigan in 1973. The Lord saved her in 1982 and filled her with the Holy Spirit on January 13, 1983. In 1985, she was called into the ministry. As she totally sold out to God, He blessed her with the gifts of intercession, discernment of spirits, prophecy and interpretation, the laying on of hands and the ministry of helps. The Lord also blessed her with the gift of helping people with their Christian walk and giving them a "now" word from the Lord.

She has been a member of International Gospel Center (IGC) for over thirty years. For the first fifteen years, she was under the leadership of the late Apostle Charles O.

Miles. She has been under the leadership of current Pastor Marvin N. Miles for the past nineteen years. She is the Supervisor of the Prayer Line Ministry, Junior Pastor, member of the Prison Ministry, Sunday School Teacher, Nursing Home Ministry team leader, Evangelist, and Nurse.

She has been married for over thirty years to Minister Dean Baker, the love of her life. They have four daughters and three grandchildren. During her Christian walk, Bonnie has received many visions and revelations from the Lord. She lives by the scriptures that say God will bless you coming in and going out and He will make you the head and not the tail.

The Lord has favored Bonnie with much success. She now owns her own company, Flash Mortgage Corporation in Canton, Michigan. In addition, Minister Baker is a Notary Public and owns four other companies.

Bonnie travels to various states preaching the Word of God, declaring that Jesus saves and will save and free you if given the opportunity. Nothing is impossible with God if you allow Him into your heart.

Author Contact
Bonnie Baker
P.O. Box 871267
Canton, MI 48187

Her first book, *Then and Now*, received a very special acknowl-edgment. In October of 2015, a group of Christian Living Books' authors, their family and friends visited our nation's capital to celebrate the distinct honor and privilege of their works being selected by the Library of Congress for inclusion in their permanent collections.

They came together from all over the country and some from the Bahamas. President Obama, Washington, D.C. Mayor Muriel Bowser, Bahamian Consul General, and respec-tive members of the House of Representatives all wrote let-ters to these authors and their publisher to commemorate and celebrate the distinction. They had a wonderful time fellowshipping, laughing with Joe Recca (the funniest man in clean comedy), being blessed by gifted singers, and taking a world class tour of D.C. Visiting the Library of Congress really solidified what an honor the selection is. The largest, most prestigious library in the world has honored men and women who love God and are committed to resourcing the Kingdom in their respective areas of influence. The Library is so awesome and beautiful that the entire experience was

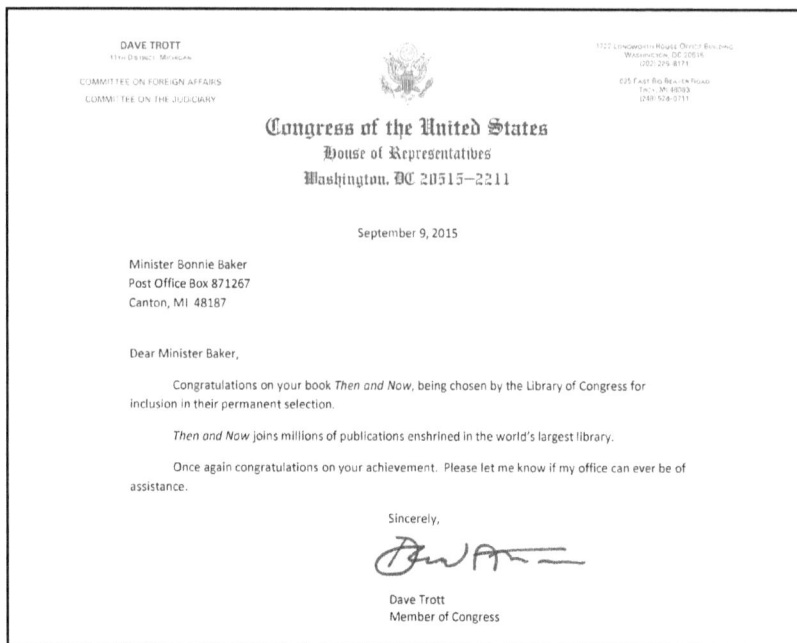

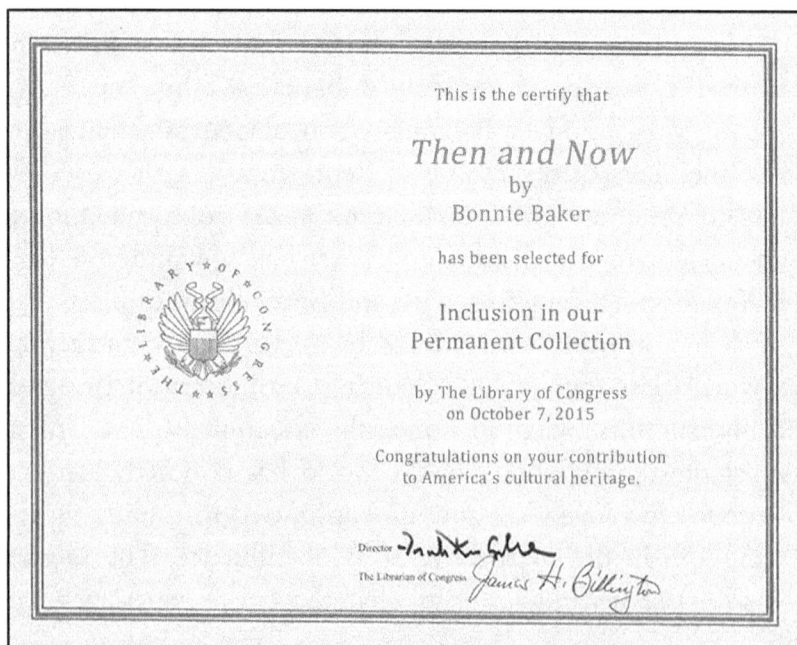

just humbling. As long as the earth remains, those works will be there, enshrined, as a part of the cultural landscape. To God be the glory for the things He has done.

THEN AND NOW

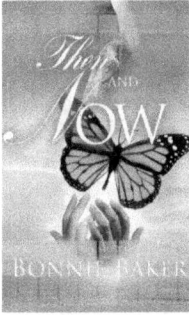

Bonnie had tasted everything the devil could serve up – alcohol, drugs, money, gambling, abuse, jail time, depression, even several encounters with death. Yet her life has taken a 180-degree turn, thanks to God and intercessory prayer. *Then and Now* is the true account of God's power to deliver us from the bondage of evil. It is sure to encourage you as you see a perfect example of God the Potter transforming a tattered life into a beautiful work of art, free from the enemy. God can free you too. He can ward off all attacks of the enemy, past, present and future. There is nothing too big for God to handle. So, whatever you are facing, trust Him and see what He can do in your life. To God be the glory.
Paperback ISBN 9781562292249   eBook ISBN 9781562298203

SURVIVING YOUR WORST FEAR

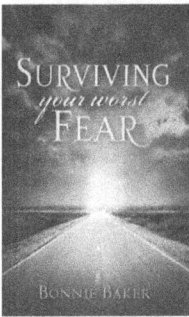

Many of us are bound by fear and don't know why – fear of the unknown, fear of not being loved, fear of heights, fear of dying, fear of failure, fear of rejection. But God didn't intend for His children to live their lives in fear. Fear opens the door for the enemy's attacks on your soul. Minister Baker shares the fears that gripped her life for years, including a debilitating fear of water following a childhood near-drowning episode. She offers the keys to divine deliverance from every fear that keeps you bound. Yes, you *can* conquer your fears!

Paperback ISBN 9781562292119   eBook ISBN 9781562292256

THEN AND NOW - PART II

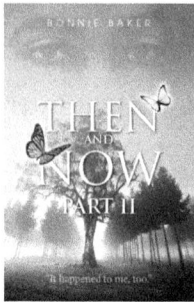

Ten years ago, Bonnie Baker penned her incredible life story. That bestselling book touched the hearts of thousands who testified, "It happened to me, too." There was much Bonnie did not tell. *Then and Now – Part 2* continues Bonnie's gut wrenching accounts of sexual abuse, physical abuse, substance abuse, exploitation and molestation. With unflinching honesty, Bonnie details the devastating consequences of looking for love in all the wrong places. Bonnie's story does not end there. NOW, Bonnie is healed, delivered, empowered and preaching the gospel. *Then and Now – Part 2* is a perfect example of God the Potter transforming a broken life into a beautiful work of art. You, too, can tell your story. Allow Bonnie's story to invoke you to get up, to turn around, to reach out to an ever-present God. He will set you on your NOW path, too.

Paperback ISBN 9781562298180   eBook ISBN 9781562298203

www.ingramcontent.com/pod-product-compliance
Lightning Source LLC
LaVergne TN
LVHW051159080426
835508LV00021B/2707